SIX WHITE DOVES & ONE PINK ROSE
A Collection of Prayers & Poems

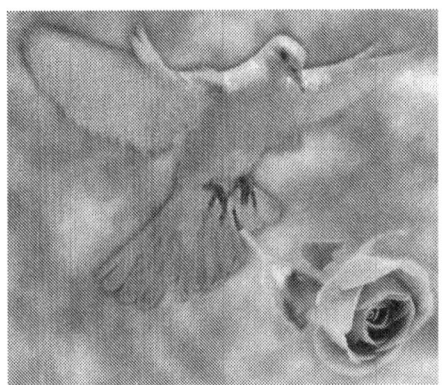

BY JOSEPHINE BROWN

"One million people commit suicide every year."
The World Health Organization

SIX WHITE DOVES &
ONE PINK ROSE

All rights reserved, no part of this publication may be reproduced by any means, electronic, mechanical photocopying, documentary, film or in any other format without prior written permission of the publisher.

>Published by
>Chipmunkapublishing
>PO Box 6872
>Brentwood
>Essex CM13 1ZT
>United Kingdom

http://www.chipmunkapublishing.com

Copyright © Josephine Brown 2007

Proof-read by John Matthews

JOSEPHINE BROWN

SIX WHITE DOVES & ONE PINK ROSE

SECOND EDITION

I write for ordinary people whose lives have been affected by tragic circumstances. I write for the many disabled people and the discrimination they silently have to endure. I write with compassion and a certain knowledge that there is a light at the end of each pathway. I know because I've been there too. If I can come through it - then so can you !

God Bless… Josephine

SIX WHITE DOVES &
ONE PINK ROSE

JOSEPHINE BROWN

Contents

1. My Prayer
2. The Rosary
3. I Cannot See, But I Can Feel
4. I Cannot Hear, But I Can See
5. Six White Doves & One Pink Rose
6. Peace Not War
7. Humility
8. I Met God On the Highway
9. When The Earth is No More
10. Please Save a Place in Heaven For Me
11. But Still I Rise
12. I Walked The Streets Of London
13. Courageously Received
14. He Touched My Heart
15. Belief
16. Final Hour

SIX WHITE DOVES &
ONE PINK ROSE

17. Sacrifice

18. Time of Take

19. What You Alone Can Achieve

20. AIDS

21. Heroin

22. Dreams & Fears

23. I Walk The Steps to Heaven

24. Prayer Before Op

25. My Mum, My World

26. Single Mum's Wish

27. I Pray To Thee This Night

28. Love & Support For Every Race

29. Big Louie

30. For The Love Of My Children

JOSEPHINE BROWN

My Prayer

My prayer is just a little prayer
I ask of thee tonight
To give me strength and courage
To battle on with all my might..

To fight the pains of life
If only for awhile
To have upon my face
A warm and friendly smile..

As there are many others
For which I pray to thee
I pray tonight for them also
Not only just for me…

**SIX WHITE DOVES &
ONE PINK ROSE**

JOSEPHINE BROWN

The Rosary
(Upon Visiting the homeless)

Take this Rosary of mine, it is all I have to give
For I am dying on this day. I fear I may not live
I have lived my past out on the streets
I have wandered through life's span
I have sung songs with the Salvation Army
I have given all that I can
The only thing I kept hanging over me, was this,
my last and loved possession.
It was my Rosary…

The winter nights have taken their toll, how the wind does howl
I can no longer tell, a tall fictitious tale
The wind is blowing the snow is so cold, its cutting into me
Please someone come forward and
Take my Rosary…

A young man stepped forward, he knelt by my side
He wiped the passing snow from my face, as my eyes felt so red and sore
I'm sure in life I had seen this man somewhere else before

He then took a blanket and covered it over me
He took my only loved possession

He took my Rosary..

SIX WHITE DOVES &
ONE PINK ROSE

JOSEPHINE BROWN

I CANNOT SEE, BUT
I CAN FEEL

I can feel the sun, but cannot see its light
I can feel the coolness of the darkening night
I cannot see flowers, but enjoy their sweet perfume
I cannot see music being played, but have enjoyed so many a happy tune..

I cannot see others, but feel their presence near
I cannot see them speak, but hear their voice so clear
I cannot see a thing, but have never felt very sad
As I can feel so much and for that I'm truly glad
I am thankful for my feelings for they shall never die
I do sometimes feel unhappy, although I cannot cry..

For when I cry, I cry inside, in my world of shadowed light but
I know that I can feel and that somehow compensates for my lack of sight

I can feel if I am loved, but cannot see my lover
I have never seen my father, nor in fact, my mother, but
I can feel them with me every moment of the day
I can listen patiently to every word they have to say..

SIX WHITE DOVES & ONE PINK ROSE

I can feel compassion for all the world's mankind
I can feel so much, even though I'm blind.

JOSEPHINE BROWN

I CANNOT HEAR, BUT I CAN SEE

I cannot hear the rain or the falling snow, but I can see and understand, much more than you know
I cannot hear, but I can see the plight of others near
I also see their negativity and of course their fears..

People repeat words to me many, many, times until I'm completely bereft
I try to tell them I can see and am not daft because
I'm deaf
My deafness brings me silent thoughts
My eyes may fill with tears
I can see and understand you know, although I cannot hear..

To hear the sound of music would bring joys to me unknown
To hear perhaps my loved ones waiting to speak to me on the telephone..

People holler and scream at me and I feel I want to laugh
For if they could see their faces, the embarrassment would last..

I'm lonely in my world of silence, so lonely its untrue but, I thank my friends and family, as much

SIX WHITE DOVES &
ONE PINK ROSE

love I feel for you
I dream one day of being able to hear, to express
myself loud and clear
That there is no need to shout at me
As I can't hear, but I can see…

JOSEPHINE BROWN

SIX WHITE DOVES & ONE PINK ROSE

Upon the ***FIRST*** day the sun did shine
A white dove flew over the earth for mankind
The ***SECOND*** day came, the sunset had risen
A light shone abundantly clear
A white dove flew over the sunset to wash away mankind's tears..
The ***THIRD*** day, a poor man was passing a valley
A benevolent sight to behold
A white dove flew over this man, his name in the Bible is foretold..
The ***FOURTH*** day the valley was echoing sweet songs from the birds that were gathering by a shaded
branch. For the tree was huge and bold
A white dove flew over the birds
It flew for the sick and the old..
The ***FIFTH*** day came and angels were adorning
throwing petals from the sky
A white dove flew over them
Giving love to our father on high..
The ***SIXTH*** day arrived and Christ could be seen
with children at his side
A white dove flew past him
Giving forgiveness to all sinners and those who had lied..
The ***SEVENTH*** day was special for this was the day
the world could sleep
A pink rose was given to mankind
A rose they would treasure and keep
For the hearts of others upon this day will always

SIX WHITE DOVES &
ONE PINK ROSE

be held in great esteem
A verse written for mankind
A verse written from a wonderful dream..

JOSEPHINE BROWN

PEACE NOT WAR
(Written before the conflict in Iraq)

Pensive thoughts of a year passing
World events procuring
Disillusionment and fear
The ultimate courage of others
God's message to the world is clear

Take not your armies
Take not your shields
Give thoughts to resolving with
words of conterminous calm
All Nations will evoke
Containment to disarm

Place no sword upon thy enemies
Show latitude instead of adversity
Let peace and love replace
A world of arrogance and farcicality..

**SIX WHITE DOVES &
ONE PINK ROSE**

JOSEPHINE BROWN

HUMILITY

I have known humility
I have known suffering and pain
I have suffered the ultimate
To have become reborn again
I watch the stars
I watch the earth collide
I watch with infinite wisdom
The pathway where exists no time
All barriers of life foretold
All strife and war unknown
I think today, is now the day that
I am going home..

SIX WHITE DOVES & ONE PINK ROSE

JOSEPHINE BROWN

I MET GOD ON THE HIGHWAY

We travelled along the highway
The road was long and hard
We'd run out of money
We'd played our final card

We passed endless miles of freeway
The sun was shining down
In my heart I knew
That only God could see us through..

Night time was falling
The air grew grey and cold
I looked across at my little girl
Who was only six years old

I had no money to buy a meal, but
God was on my mind
A little old man walked up to me
I saw that he was blind..

I asked if I could give him a ride
He turned to me and said
I'll give you 20 bucks my friend, if
in your car I can lay my head,,

He slept the night in my car, by morning he had gone
On the back seat of my car - a Bible Icould see
I knew at that moment, that God had visited me..

SIX WHITE DOVES & ONE PINK ROSE

JOSEPHINE BROWN

WHEN THE EARTH IS NO MORE

When the earth is no more and the world is sleeping
A man will appear to pray for the weeping of past, present and future generations for the fathers, mothers and all relations
He will pass the place where many have died
We will pass the place where many have cried
He will pray to the father in heaven for a solution
To give the world complete absolution

He will pray for the animals, insects and birds
He will bring them forth with just a few words
He will pray for the children whose suffering was great
He will pray that these children will pass through his gates
As the garden of heaven has always been there
For the suffering generations of the world's despair

When the earth has been resurrected with help from the father
Let no man forget the world's disaster
To triumph through life
With victory in death
Is just another miracle our father has left

His teachings are simple - he wants us to love
Not fight like animals for a neighbours blood
To live is to conquer all life's ambitions

SIX WHITE DOVES & ONE PINK ROSE

Not to be proud with deep inhibitions..

To pray for the person who condemns you on sight
Pray that this person will someday walk in the light
To walk in darkness, is to walk in fear
To walk with the father, your mind becomes clear
that the angels are coming and the Lord will be here…

JOSEPHINE BROWN

PLEASE SAVE A PLACE IN HEAVEN FOR ME...

As I wander through this world
A homeless, unloved fool
Awaiting hope, that life will get better
A greater power to perhaps rule
My soul is crying out to thee
***Please, save a place in
heaven for me..***

As I walk the streets of London in the burning heat
My eyes are filled with tears because
I've got nowhere to sleep
I look towards the heavens, but I cannot see
***Please, save a place in
heaven for me..***

I feel such hunger, but have no money to eat
My legs are heavy and tired
Blood is burning my blistered feet
I've lived my life neither good nor bad, but today,
my Father,
I grow weary and sad
For there is no rest here, today, tomorrow, or
future to be

***Please, save a place in
heaven for me..***

Hungry, tired and a heart that beats no more
I enter your heavens, hungry and poor

SIX WHITE DOVES &
ONE PINK ROSE

I apologise for the state I'm in, but Father
I can now hear your angels sing
Tears are washing away my fears as I reach out to
your heavens excitedly

*To say… Thank you Father, for having
saved a place in heaven for me…*

JOSEPHINE BROWN

BUT, STILL I RISE..

You may malign, you may judge
What price to pay for ultimate love
The love a mother has for her Son
A mental illness that has now begun
To be met with such prejudice and beguiled disguise
But, Still I Rise..

To await hope, where none is to hand
To be met with the closing of doors
One after another, feelings of inferiority
As to many I'm just an unfortunate mother
The tears are there, but I do not cry
But, Still I Rise..

Hopes and dreams of a mother become shattered by others
To have been blessed with a courageous young man
The doors remain bolted and tied
One day to burst open wide
Awaiting this child to fly
But, Still I Rise..

Cruel words I endure and receive
Inner feelings I neither deny or believe that the mentally ill will one day, not be
perceived as evil and vile
The arrival of arrogance, mischief and lies
Yesterday, today and tomorrow
A heart that is filled only with compassionate pride

SIX WHITE DOVES & ONE PINK ROSE

I remain, hopeful, yet fearful of the future years
Expecting only heartache, ridicule and an abundance of tears
But. Still I Rise..

JOSEPHINE BROWN

I WALKED THE STREETS OF LONDON..
(Written after the death of Princess Diana)

I walked the streets of London upon a cold November day
My hands tucked in my pockets for that is where they'll stay
I had walked this way many times as a small child
These streets of London I had so adored
I paused to rest, my thoughts running wild, engulfed with half rage and scorn
For the past seemed an eternity awaiting a future less tethered and torn
For all the riches in this world could never enhance more freely
Than the spirit that binds us all, like hunger
The future is locked within the past like the eloquence of light
That shines beneath the shaded trees amidst the secrets of eternal life
I walked the streets of London, inconspicuously happy, alone yet out of sight..

SIX WHITE DOVES & ONE PINK ROSE

JOSEPHINE BROWN

COURAGEOUSLY RECEIVED

A career within a notable profession
Acceptance of perhaps, a University Degree
Injuries in life that were suffered, would not allow
this to become reality
All these achievements are great, until you begin
to equate
Forgiveness from within, you have to now
negotiate..

The magic of writing poetry which can allow others
a differing point of view.
Because of the written words in life – alternate
pathways we can pursue..

It isn't what you have achieved in life
It's how you feel inside
The difference between walking with your head
held down, or walking through life
with pride..

To know you have won a battle
A battle to succeed
A certificate you have earned in life and have at
last, courageously received..

SIX WHITE DOVES &
ONE PINK ROSE

JOSEPHINE BROWN

HE TOUCHED MY HEART..

There was a garden in the sky with flowers everywhere
I walked along the pathway
In my mind I felt happy and gay
I wanted to speak to God, as I had plenty to say
I asked, if I could stay in his garden
God turned to me and said
"You will come to the garden again my child, as you are truly blessed".

I am now in a place full of wonder and peace
Where angels were calling my name
I soon came to realise that life for me, had become spiritually changed

The pathways of life can be difficult, we know, but this is the way our spirituality must grow
To become to others a friend in times of need
Is the first spiritual sowing of an infinite seed

God placed his hand upon my head and I found myself back in my hospital bed
He touched my heart, he healed my wounds of life
Today, I most certainly met our Lord Jesus Christ..

SIX WHITE DOVES &
ONE PINK ROSE

JOSEPHINE BROWN

BELIEF

A man who has wealth has power in this life

This is believed..

A man who has love in his heart, has but eternal life in the next

In thee we trust..

A man who has sinned, a murderer, or thief
To have said sorry from the heart, will truly be blessed

In thee we know..

A man whose betrayed those who had his trust
Can only be forgiven from heaven above

Thy Will, be done..

Be at peace with yourself, with your family and friends
For it is those who will forgive you and whose love you can depend

In his names sake…

SIX WHITE DOVES &
ONE PINK ROSE

JOSEPHINE BROWN

FINAL HOUR

My eyes grow dim
My mind is unclear
O holy father, please be near

My heart is ready to enter eternity
My body approaches with uncertainty

As the tear of death in my final hour does arrive
I see angels gathered by my side

I glance once more at the world
I've known
As I cease my life
I feel not alone

To enter your heavens, I feel not afraid
As in my life, my debts I've paid

I may be entering another world unknown to me,
but my eyes are
still strong and I can truly see

I leave this poem for others to see
That there is no death – just a new life in eternity..

SIX WHITE DOVES & ONE PINK ROSE

JOSEPHINE BROWN

SACRIFICE

Happiness is, but a state of mind
Sadness, is equally the same
Misguided values of mankind are truly to blame

To sacrifice all that you have won't make a lot of sense
Until, like I, you come to realise that a good heart is worth more than
any money spent…

SIX WHITE DOVES &
ONE PINK ROSE

JOSEPHINE BROWN

TIME OF TAKE..

This time of today where people fear to live
In this world of take as much as you can and never think to give
A world that is governed by an "inflation rate"

This is a time, a time of take

People who steal, cheat and lie
Hit old folk until they die
Law doesn't seem to worry them or even make them care.
They live to hurt other people's lives and cause their victims so much anger and hate

Yes, this truly is a time, a time of not give, but take..

A man lies bleeding by the gutter - most walk past with an inconsequential utter
Thinking only of themselves, they pretend they've just gone blind.
In their heart they're guilty, its left only in their mind..

The memory of what they have witnessed
They really cannot shake

Yes, this truly is a time, a time of not give, but take...

SIX WHITE DOVES & ONE PINK ROSE

JOSEPHINE BROWN

WHAT YOU ALONE CAN ACHIEVE…
(Written for all 'battered wives' everywhere; including myself)

I had a violent husband, couldn't stand life anymore
The pain each day I suffered when I would hit the floor
My mouth was always bleeding, my mind was shattered so
I packed my case and left, but I'd nowhere else to go
For many years I tried to show him that violence cannot win
Now I must tread a different pathway
A new life to begin..

My childhood was no better
No physical contact had I known, but I say to others
sincerely, it does no good to moan
Pick up the fragments of your life
Go forward and believe
As you would be surprised, just what you alone can achieve..

SIX WHITE DOVES &
ONE PINK ROSE

JOSEPHINE BROWN

AIDS

Sitting alone in a darkened room
Realising that I could die soon
My thoughts are muddled and unclear
My soul is crying out with fear

I want my friends to call and help
To encourage my mind with a little hope
My friends have run away from me
O God, how do I cope?

There is so much I want to achieve
I have little in this world to leave
Except for the following words I've come to believe

To hope, is to achieve
To achieve, is to conquer
To help others becomes a solution
In God there is, absolution

Can someone, anyone help to ease my pain?
O God I pray to thee
Please give me the courage to face life, once again..

.

SIX WHITE DOVES & ONE PINK ROSE

JOSEPHINE BROWN

HEROIN
(Written on behalf of all mothers whose children are affected by drug addiction)

Twisting and turning, not knowing what to do
My child is sick with heroin, he has bitten off, more than he can chew
My child when born was beautiful, happy and so secure
Now he's twisted up inside, with eyes of fire and very obscure

What is this hell I'm being put through
My heart is sad for I'm trying to reach him, but alas I don't know what to do.

His emotions are fierce and I'm afraid of this
How I miss those tender moments when all would be well with just one kiss..

I should never be able to tell of my life now
This inner most hell
For I can see my beloved son ending up in a solitary police cell
Sitting silently, as if no more, until that is, he hit's the floor

How do I live with this?
How do I make him to resist?
Have I failed him as a mother?
As we cannot now even touch each other

Each day that passes, makes me cringe

SIX WHITE DOVES & ONE PINK ROSE

Will I, I wonder, find yet another syringe
Will he holler, scream and shout, or will he strike me with a clout
Will he watch my every move
Or will he cry and shall I soothe
Will he shake, or my money take, or will I just cry inside
Perhaps, my son will stare at me
A stare that makes me want to hide
Will my once bonny lad, ever truly be sane
O God, I pray to thee, please help me have my son back once again….

JOSEPHINE BROWN

DREAMS AND FEARS

I walked along the seashore
My life had been difficult and unsure
My days remained at a steady pace
Belief in myself I didn't want to face

I came across a badly dressed boy
I thought he must be very poor
We talked together whilst watching the waves on the edge of this seashore

He told me he was all alone
No one to help him, no one of his very own
I couldn't give him money
I couldn't give him food
I could only give him my friendship
His eyes began to fill with tears
As we walked together talking about all our dreams and fears

We laughed together, he told me about his life of sin, but no money or food could I give him
We forgot about eating or money
We enjoyed ourselves, it was really funny
We gave each other what we needed most of all
To believe in this world
To have stood together united
To have stood together so tall…

SIX WHITE DOVES & ONE PINK ROSE

JOSEPHINE BROWN

I WALK THE STEPS TO HEAVEN..

In the quiet of the night giving the rising of the morning sun
Life has now fulfilled its meaning
It is now, although inconsequential to others,
Life has now begun

Forgotten are the sorrows
Forgotten are the memories that have kept my mind in the tragic past
I now walk the steps to heaven where my eternal life will truly start

I wander through the heavens
In the quiet of the earthly night
I'm filled with wondrous feelings
Feelings of heartfelt delight

I've been welcomed by many others whom I haven't seen for years
Death is, but for a moment
There is no need for tears

Money isn't an issue I'm truly glad to say
Heaven is for everyone where you never have to pay

Any debts or sins you may have incurred are left indeed, behind, never again to be
I now walk the steps to heaven where illness

SIX WHITE DOVES &
ONE PINK ROSE

disappears and where all the blind can see..

JOSEPHINE BROWN

PRAYER BEFORE OP..

O Lord in heaven, as we've been friends for years
I'm fearful of my operation, I've shed so many tears
I can't write much longer, as I don't feel very alert
My arms are packed with needles, they really do quite hurt
I don't wish to sound morbid or dreary, but you say
in your good book, which makes more sense than mere theory
"If thy body offends thee, then cut the offending part off"
Well, my Lord, as you can see - its jolly well all I've got!
Blessed angels in the sky, I further pray this night, that
whilst you are about it, could you please restore my sight
I'll give up my smoking, I'll do everything you ask
As I don't quite fancy the alternative, to be buried beneath the grass
Should you O Lord, require my presence in your heavens so bright, but old
Could you, O holy father see that I am never cold ?

SIX WHITE DOVES &
ONE PINK ROSE

JOSEPHINE BROWN

MY MUM, MY WORLD

I had a courageous mother who gave her love to me and when I was in trouble, she would sit me upon her knee
One night as I lay sleeping in my little bed
An angel came from heaven to say my mum was dead

I woke up early the next morning to see if it was true
My mum had gone to heaven as the angel had told me so
One day we'll be together and keep the love we had, but until then, dear mum, I shall be so very sad

To think we could have had longer, like man people do
I wish you would come back mum, as I really do miss you
This world is such an empty world without your loving touch
I think your going to heaven was really a bit too much

You have been so very brave to face the end alone
Especially in good cheer
I hope the day that I go to heaven, that I too, will have no fear
I say farewell dear mum

SIX WHITE DOVES &
ONE PINK ROSE

No more tears shall I weep
As I have so many happy memories
That I shall always treasure and keep..

JOSEPHINE BROWN

SINGLE MUM'S WISH

I am a single mum and happy though I am
It would be nice to meet one day, an honest reliable man
I love my children lots and lots, but I've not had a good night out since they were tiny tots
I'd like to go shopping, completely on my own
No children allowed, not even a mobile phone
I'd like to lie in bed, just for one whole day
I'd then go out in the evening and dance the night away
One day, I hope, I'll get my wish
One day, it will come true – but no matter what happens within my life
I say to you my children, I'll always have love and time for you..

SIX WHITE DOVES & ONE PINK ROSE

JOSEPHINE BROWN

I PRAY TO THEE
THIS NIGHT

I pray for humanity the ill and the blind
I pray that humanity will become wiser and kind
I pray for sick animals, insects and birds
That the heavenly father will heal with just a few words

I pray this night for peace to reign
I pray goodness and mercy will shine once again

I pray for the many who are mentally ill
I pray their minds will be cured at God's will
I pray for the many who have lost sight of love
I pray they may be guided by the angels above

I pray for all people who have been victims of crime
I pray that God will bring peace to all nations
creating a greater understanding for all of mankind

SIX WHITE DOVES &
ONE PINK ROSE

JOSEPHINE BROWN

LOVE AND SUPPORT FOR EVERY RACE

Hopes and dreams that fade into space
Love and support for every race
For the many people who do not want to go on
I say to them be courageous and strong

You have a right to this world
You have the right to live
Say to your oppressors
Its now time to forgive

The old regimes to be cast aside
To walk with confidence and never to hide
For whatever is happening in your life today
I would just like to say

There are many who cannot stand, speak, have sight, nor can walk with pride

To have remembered that is ..

The words of another
"But for the Grace of God, there Go I"

SIX WHITE DOVES &
ONE PINK ROSE

JOSEPHINE BROWN

BIG LOUIE
A Soldier of courage who was killed in Iraq.

The night before big Louie was killed, he joked
and laughed and snored as he slept
This big hearted guy who'd fought and prevented
many a crime
Life for big Louie was unknowingly, running out of
time

This gentle giant, this soldier of pride
He fought bravely in Iraq with his mates by his
side
Stuart, his friend, by night and by day
Never believed big Louie would be blown away

This brave soldier, big Louie, like many, will be
remembered for courage, tenacity and duty call
As this was a soldier who'd won the love and
respect of his Country and had become loved by
all

Farewell, big Louie, our hero, our friend that we
were blessed to know and love
Farewell, big Louie, as you enter God's heavens
above

We will hear you laugh mate, we will hear you joke
For you are, and always will be within our hearts
big Louie,
Our friend, our soldier of courage, and a
wonderful bloke.

SIX WHITE DOVES & ONE PINK ROSE

JOSEPHINE BROWN

FOR THE LOVE OF MY CHILDREN

Don't cry for me, my children
For I shall always be by your side
The angels here in heaven
Will gladly be my guides

As I walk beside you
I will hear your prayers at night
I know, one day we will meet again
Have faith, and you'll see I'm right

I will watch your smiling faces
As you triumph through your years
I hope, my loves, my darlings
You will not have any fears

The heavens are now my home
With stars shining bright and gay
Do not be sad, my children for I'll not leave you for one day

Your thoughts and all the hopes you have
Will be thoughts held dear to me
I've not really left you
I am, but a closer walk with thee..

www.ingramcontent.com/pod-product-compliance
Ingram Content Group UK Ltd.
Pitfield, Milton Keynes, MK11 3LW, UK
UKHW041413180426
11947UKWH00007B/104

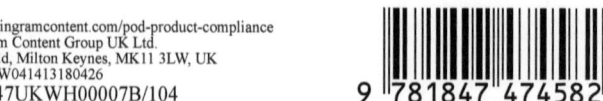